Obesity Code And Management; Unlocking The Ultimate Code For Weight Loss Naturally

Jamie P.Louis

Table of contents

Table of contents

Chapter 1

The epidemic's "obesity" source

Obesity is a well-known pandemic that is impacting people all around the world. Despite several attempts and suggestions to reduce the incidence of obesity and its co-morbidities, this epidemic has been occurring more often since the 1980s. The root reasons for obesity have been identified, and they are mostly connected to a genetic sensitivity to put on weight as a result of increased calorie intake and decreased energy expenditures, as well as an environmental propensity to do so. Furthermore, since the 1980s, many structural environmental changes have produced an obesogenic environment marked by the availability of high-calorie, low-quality food, and little physical exercise. All of this leads to increased body weight gain and a global public health problem not only a distinct patient's disease that generally fails to respond to diets and increased activity

In those who are genetically predisposed to obesity, fried food consumption has to be restricted since it may interact with genes related to fat.

Healthy lifestyles can mitigate the consequences of these so-called "obesity genes" since many people who possess them do not become overweight. In this article, the effects of genes and gene-environment interactions on the development of obesity are briefly discussed.

Obesity is a health issue in the twenty-first century that affects both rich and poor, educated and illiterate, Westernized and non-Westernized societies. The so-called "fat mass and obesity-associated" (FTO) gene on chromosome 16 has the first obesity-related gene variations. People who possess one of these very frequent gene variations have a 20–30% increased risk of obesity than those who do not. On chromosome 18, near to the melanocortin-4 receptor gene, researchers discovered the second obesity-related gene variation (the same gene responsible for a rare form of monogenic obesity).

New polymorphisms or mutations take a very long time to propagate. What then has changed over the past 40 years of increased obesity rates if our genes have essentially remained the same? Our environment, which includes the physical, social, political, and economic factors affecting our activity levels and dietary habits. The current increase in overweight and obesity has been significantly attributed to environmental changes that make it simpler for people to overeat and more difficult for them to engage in adequate physical exercise.

The gene-environment connections that affect obesity is still in its early stages. According to my research thus far, having so-called "obesity genes" does not automatically lead to becoming overweight in most cases. Instead, it appears that eating a balanced diet and exercising regularly may reduce part of the risk of obesity that is tied to genes. Depending on their family history and ethnicity, the majority of people likely have some inherited susceptibility to obesity. Changes in nutrition, lifestyle, or other environmental variables are typically necessary to go from a hereditary susceptibility to obesity itself. These are a few of the alteration.

On chromosome 16, the "fat mass and obesity-associated" (FTO) gene has the first obesity-related gene variations. These gene variations are quite common, and those who possess one have an increased risk of obesity of 20 to 30% compared to those who do not. On chromosome 18, near the melanocortin-4 receptor gene, the second obesity-related gene variation has been discovered (the same gene responsible for a rare form of monogenic obesity).

Research on the gene-environment connections that affect obesity is still in its early stages. According to the research thus far, having so-called "obesity genes" does not automatically lead to becoming overweight in most cases. Instead, it appears that eating a balanced diet and exercising regularly may reduce part of the risk of obesity that is tied to genes.

Depending on their family history and ethnicity, the majority of people likely have some inherited susceptibility to obesity. Changes in nutrition, lifestyle, or other environmental variables are typically necessary to go from a hereditary susceptibility to obesity itself. These are a few of the alterations:

The easy access to food at all hours of the day and in locations that previously did not sell food, such as gas stations, pharmacies, and office supply stores; a sharp decline in physical activity during work, household chores, and free time, especially among children; an increase in the amount of time spent watching television, using computers, and engaging in other sedentary activities; and the proliferation of highly processed foods, fast food, and beverages with added sugars.

Physiology, development, and adaptation in humans are all influenced by genes. No one is exempt from obesity. Yet surprisingly little is understood about the precise genes that cause obesity and the scope of so-called "genetic environment interactions," the intricate connections between our ancestry and our upbringing.

Chapter 2

Momentum and a new diet

If you want to lose weight, the optimal times to consume breakfast, lunch, and supper are.
When it comes to weight loss, the time you select to eat might be really important.
Many of us fail to consider other elements, such as the ideal time to eat breakfast, lunch, and supper since weight loss advice frequently focuses so heavily on what to eat to lose weight.

Early in the morning, namely around 7.11 am, is the optimal time to eat breakfast. Additionally, it's best to eat your lunch between 12.30 and 1 pm rather than later. The optimal timing is at 12:38. Additionally, the later you have dinner, the worse it may be for your diet. Try to have supper between 6 and 6.30 p.m.; the study found that 6.14 p.m. was ideal. However, if you wake up later than usual and can't imagine preparing a nutritious breakfast before the sun rises, it regulates our hunger hormones and keeps us fuller and content for longer.

Your eating period is "all about balance. It makes sense to spread out your food intake for the remaining meals of the day to sustain energy. If your schedule permits, try to keep to a 1 pm luncheon and a 6 pm dinnertime since our bodies respond strongly to the pattern. Meals that are delayed until the late afternoon or evening may lead to overeating or poor dietary decisions."

What time of day is ideal for snacking?
The ideal times to have snacks are around 11.01 am,
3.14 pm, and 9.31 pm. At this point, you are most
vulnerable to losing your willpower. Anytime you go
more than four hours without meals or just after a hard
activity, you should think about taking a snack.

However, not all of your go-to snacks will satisfy you in
between meals, so it's vital to pick wisely. Select foods
with high protein content and high fiber content to help
you feel fuller for longer. Even while snacking, it's crucial
to always eat mindfully. Stay alert and at the moment.
To help you make and keep healthier dietary decisions,
plan your meals and healthy snacks in advance. While
eating a high-protein diet it might be a fantastic decision
in some circumstances, it's important to watch how
much protein you consume while trying to feel full. Avoid
consuming too much protein at once, especially if it is
combined with little to no fiber, advises the author. Any
excess is made accessible to our gut microorganisms
because there is always a limit to how much our body
can absorb. Although our gut microorganisms prefer
high-fiber diets, if none are present, they will begin to
degrade any undigested protein. This procedure may
result in goods that are bad for lifespan and intestinal
health.

What guideline is the most crucial when trying to lose
weight?

The most crucial thing to keep in mind if you want to lose weight is that you need to eat fewer calories each day than you burn. Unfortunately, this is the only method to lose weight. It is known as an energy deficit or a calorie deficit, and it may be accomplished in a variety of ways. Although low-carb, high-fat diets like the Banting diet and the 16:8 plan may advertise themselves as certain ways to lose weight, you won't notice any results unless you're in this deficit.

This is due to the fact that when you eat, your body uses the nutrients it contains to produce energy. The body needs this energy for everything from breathing to moving. If you consume more calories than your body requires, you will have surplus energy, which will eventually turn into fat. You won't have enough energy if you consume less than you need, and your body will start using its fat reserves as fuel. Weight loss occurs during the latter step.

What is the damage of skipping meals?
Never, under any circumstances, skip meals.
It has been shown that skipping breakfast is linked to a number of unhealthy indicators, including weight gain and altered glucose metabolism. According to many, having breakfast reduces impulsive snacking and helps set the tone for a healthy diet throughout the day. Your metabolism may be set up for the day by having a well-balanced breakfast that includes high-fiber foods like berries and a decent supply of protein, such as Greek yogurt.

View from above of a gray rural table with a mango banana smoothie bowl with natural greek yogurt, chia seeds, and a healthy vegetarian dessert with honey (Mango banana smoothie bowl with natural greek yogurt, chia seeds, and)

But folks don't only like to skip breakfast. The second most popular meal to skip was dinner, with up to 57% of respondents doing so. Those who skipped lunch or supper were more likely to be overweight, which has repercussions beyond just weight gain. Men and women who skipped their final meal of the day were more likely to get less sleep at night, which contributed to feelings of constant fatigue. Additionally, they were more likely to be strong drinkers or smokers.

You should enter a calorie deficit in addition to eating breakfast, lunch, and supper at the recommended times. Take a look at a calorie counter to determine yours. this will inform you of your maintenance level and shortfall threshold. For instance, if you're a 30-year-old woman who is 5 feet 4 inches tall and weighs 70 kilograms (the average weight for people in the UK), your daily calorie goal to lose 0.25 kilograms per week will be 1,677 calories.

After crossing that line, your day can look like this:

Breakfast
If you can, try to achieve 400 calories with any of these low-calorie breakfast recipes.

395 calories in blackcurrant bircher muesli
A quick farmhouse fry-up contains 221 calories and 118 calories per 250 ml glass of orange juice.
Muffins from Slimming World with smoked salmon have 295 calories, while a tall coffee from Starbucks has 90 calories.

Stick to no more than 500 calories for lunch (between 12:30 and 1 pm). Halfway through the day, you'll need a boost, so it's critical to provide your body with the nutrition and protein it requires. Choose complex carbs for this instead of refined ones like those in white pasta, rice, and bread. You won't feel drained of energy a few hours after lunch and you'll stay fuller for longer.
Chicken spaghetti with peas by Ainsley Harriott has 426 calories.
Tortilla with spring vegetables: 390 calories
1 wholemeal roll and a quick Quorn lunch bowl have a combined calorie count of 155.

Dinner The evening meal, which should be eaten between 6 and 6.30 p.m., should contain about 500 calories. It's advisable to focus your meal on protein and veggies rather than opting for a spaghetti dish that is high in carbohydrates because you don't want to feel overly full before bed.
Chicken with chickpeas with mild spices: 309 calories
302 calories from peppers and spicy turkey stuffing
300 calories in a split pea and veggie curry

Don't exceed 400, 500, and 500 calories for breakfast, lunch, and supper. You'll be able to reward yourself with two 100-calorie snacks during the day if you accomplish this. Any milk you add to your tea or coffee will add an additional 77 calories to your intake.

Chapter 3

Basic strategies against obesity include meditation, exercise, and good sleep hygiene.

It's not enough to eat the right things and exercise enough to lose weight; you also need to work on your mental health. This is because your weight reduction attempts will fail if you don't adopt the proper mindset. Here are ten tips for losing weight.

1. Develop a healthy living mindset

Instead of having a weight-loss mindset, weight management is more about leading a healthy lifestyle. Establish healthy lifestyle practices and make an effort not to pay too much attention to your weight loss. Instead, concentrate on eating the correct meals and exercising sufficiently. Healthy living also entails leading a fulfilling life and taking care of your mental health. You won't be in the correct state of mind to make the right food decisions until your mind is in the right place.

2. Decide to be happy despite your current circumstances

Some people decide they won't be content until they drop a certain amount of weight or for another reason. In other words, for them to be content, they require a license. The catch-22 is that your attempts to control your weight will be thwarted by low self-esteem. You alone are responsible for your happiness. Being the person you were meant to be will go a long way toward reaching happiness, and if you achieve that, it will be easier to achieve your optimum weight. It is up to you to determine your own vocation in life.

3. Be yourself

Since no one else is like you, be the best version of yourself rather than a carbon copy of someone else. Instead of feeling jealous of individuals who are talented in other areas, it is best to develop your own special abilities and talents. You should share your talents with others so that they can benefit from them rather than hiding or hoarding them for yourself. When it comes to weight loss, trying to acquire a model-like figure when you have a different body type is pointless.

4. Don't compare yourself with others.
Run your own race, and let everyone else finish theirs. People with low self-esteem frequently compare themselves negatively to others. True, people frequently date their self-esteem. People who experience the same problems as they do draw them. Accept yourself as you are, and if people don't like you for who you are, that's their issue, not yours. Do your absolute best!

5. Take no notice of the infomercials

Advertisers will employ every available tactic to pique your interest. Making you feel bad about who you are is a part of it. When you look at some of the commercials, you can actually understand why some women's self-esteem falls. In most ads, there is a disclaimer that reads, "Results are not typical." Be aware that there are numerous more who tried their hardest but were unsuccessful for every person who appears in those testimonies. The success tales you read are frequently embellished.

6. Ignore the before and after ads
Don't pay attention to the before and after commercials. You should only be worried about your own before and after pictures. The before the picture is always an unattractive one. You have no idea what transpires to achieve the after photo's aesthetically pleasing result.

7. Make small changes daily
In order for your body to adjust to a new habit, whether it be a change in your food or a new workout regimen, make incremental modifications to your diet. Create positive habits by making small, manageable changes. Even though it will all take time, it is preferable to try to accomplish too much too quickly and then give up. Rome wasn't created in a day, and nothing worthwhile ever was, so have patience.

8. Don't lose heart

When you are not making much progress, it might be discouraging. Don't give up; if you stick to your healthy living plan, you will at least feel confident that you are acting morally. Keep your mind off your concerns by concentrating on your activities. No matter what, have fun enjoying your life.

9. Take up new hobbies and sports
This is crucial for your well-being because your attempts to manage your weight will be ineffective if you are not in the appropriate frame of mind. Do you know what "comfort eating" means? You can interact with others through the sport, which aids in expanding your network of friends and acquaintances. Participating in a sport can undoubtedly aid in maintaining your mental stability and helping you to manage your weight. You can participate in a variety of sports, regardless of how unfit you are. Better than not exercising is taking a little stroll around the block. The secret is to make exercise a habit.

10. Understand there are no magic formulas.

The secret to getting the body you want doesn't exist. You cannot lose weight by using an easy fix or a quick fix. You must choose whether the work and sacrifice are worthwhile. For every body type, there is a perfect weight. You must therefore determine what body type is best for your weight.

Exercise

A good strategy to reduce weight and keep it under control is to exercise consistently. But if you've been inactive for a long or are overweight, it might be challenging to begin a new exercise regimen. You may find it more motivating to start and continue exercising if you concentrate on its advantages. Of course, consult your doctor before beginning any workout regimen.

Advantages of consistent exercise.
It's difficult to feel good about yourself when you're out of shape. Even worse, being overweight increases your chance of getting health issues including type 2 diabetes, high blood pressure, and heart disease. The American Heart Association claims that even a small amount of weight loss can result in several health benefits. Decreasing just five to ten pounds can help lower blood pressure and lessen the burden on your heart if you are overweight.

Additionally, exercise can lower cholesterol. Exercise increases HDL cholesterol, also known as "good" cholesterol while decreasing LDL cholesterol, also known as "bad" cholesterol. Additionally, you're more likely to have a restful night's sleep, which might increase your productivity and focus.

The best part is that regular exercise improves your mood. And that helps you feel more confident.

Include regular exercise in your everyday regimen.

You don't have to start training for a half-marathon or join a gym to start an exercise regimen. To be sure you are healthy enough to start an exercise regimen, check with your doctor first. Finding methods to include physical exercise into your day is the simplest approach to start exercising:

(1) Take the stairs rather than the elevator.

(2) At the grocery shop, park far from the front door.

(3) Sit on an exercise ball while working to build back and core strength.

(4) Take a stroll after work or after lunch.

(5) Exercise while watching TV by using hand weights or resistance bands.

(6) Play some music and start dancing.

(7) Be more active to reduce weight
It's time to begin exercising if your doctor advises you to reduce weight. You'll quickly discover that regular exercise has many advantages and is well worth the effort. Follow this straightforward advice to begin exercising:

Begin gradually.

If it's been a while since you've exercised, ease into your new workout routine and give your body some time to become used to it.

Choose a task you enjoy.
Enjoy the view while you bike or stroll through a local park. As you work out on an elliptical machine, listen to podcasts.

Work out with a friend.
Being social might help you stay motivated to work out more.

Remain hydrated.
Water is important to consume before, during, and after exercise.

Occasionally switch up your training regimen.
The diversity of physical activities you engage in keeps you engaged and keeps boredom at bay.

Put on a fitness monitor.
You may establish objectives using fitness trackers and health apps. Monitoring your development can inspire you.

What level of workout is required?
You engage in strength training at least twice per week, flexibility, and stretching activities, as well as at least 150 minutes of moderate cardiovascular activity each week. Focus on workouts that are easy on your joints if

you are overweight, such as walking, swimming, or water exercises.

If 150 minutes of exercise a week sounds overwhelming, divide your workout into smaller segments. Your objective should be to exercise for 30 minutes each day, five days a week. However, you are not required to do your 30-minute workout all at once. You may exercise for only 10 minutes at a time and still get results.

If you ever have chest discomfort, shortness of breath, nausea, pain in the neck or jaw, or any type of muscle or joint pain when exercising, stop immediately.

Celebrate your achievement.
Having a motivational factor to be active makes it simpler to incorporate exercise into your daily life. Identify strategies to recognize your weight loss accomplishments. After you accomplish a goal, get new exercise equipment. Or, once you drop five pounds, treat yourself to a massage. Just watch out that your incentives don't conflict with your objectives.

Chapter 4

Conclusion

1200 Calorie Weight Loss Diet Chart Plan

The components of the optimum diet chart may be discussed in great detail. One's dietary needs, however, vary depending on many things. It could vary based on gender, for instance, as male and female nutritional needs are different.

Geographical factors may also be at play because the cuisines of North and South India differ significantly. Since a vegetarian or vegan consumes food quite differently from a non-vegetarian, meal choices become important in this situation.

However, we have created a diet strategy that is great for losing weight while eating Indian food. This sample 7-day diet plan, commonly known as a 1200-calorie diet plan, is for educational purposes only and should not be used by anybody without first visiting a nutritionist.

Day 1 of the weight loss diet plan chart

Have oat porridge with mixed nuts for breakfast after starting the day with cucumber water.
Lunch will thereafter be a roti with dal and gajar matar sabzi.

Dinner will be dal and lauki sabzi with roti after that.
Dietary Plan for Day 1
6:30 AM Detox Water with Cucumber (1 glass)
8:00 AM Porridge with Oats and Skim Milk (1 bowl)

Various Nuts (25 grams)
Midnight Slightly Skimmed Paneer (100 grams)
2:00 PM Vegetable Salad, Variety (1 katori)
2:10 PM The Sabzi Gajar Matar
4:00 PM sliced fruit (1 cup) Buttermilk (1 glass) (1 glass)
5:30 PM Tea with Less Milk and Sugar (1 teacup)
8:50 PM Vegetable Salad, Variety

Day 2 of the diet plan for weight loss
Eat a stuffed roti with mixed vegetables and curd for
breakfast on the second day.
Have half a katori of methi rice and lentil curry for lunch.
Then, finish your day with green chutney and sautéed
vegetables.
Day 2 Nutrition Plan
6:30 AM Detox Water with Cucumber (1 glass)
8:00 AM Curd Roti With Mixed Veggies Stuffed In (2
pieces)
Noon Slightly Skimmed Paneer (100 grams)
2:00 PM Vegetable Salad, Variety (1 katori)
2:10 PM Linguine Curry (0.75 bowl) Curry Rice
4:00 PM 0.5 tiny (2-3/4″ dia.) apple Buttermilk (1 glass)
(1 glass)
5:30 PM less sugar, milk, and coffee (0.5 teacups)
8:50 PM Salad of Mixed Vegetables (1 katori)

9:00 PM Vegetables in a Sauté with Paneer 1 roti and 1 chapati
a green relish (2 tablespoons)

Day 3 of the diet plan for weight loss
On day 3, breakfast would consist of yogurt made with skim milk and multigrain toast.
Have paneer, sautéed veggies, and some green chutney in the afternoon.
To make sure you conclude the day on a healthy note, eat half a katori of methi rice and some lentil curry.
Diet Plan for Day Three
6:30 AM Detox Water with Cucumber (1 glass)
8:00 AM Yogurt made with skim milk, 1 cup (8 fl oz)
Granular Toast (2 toast)
Noon Slightly Skimmed Paneer (100 grams)
2:00 PM Vegetable Salad, Variety (1 katori)
2:10 PM Vegetables in a Sauté with Paneer Green Chutney (2 tablespoons)

4:00 PM Banana (0.5 tiny; 6-7/8" to 6" long) Buttermilk (1 glass) (1 glass)
5:30 PM Tea with Less Milk and Sugar (1 teacup)
8:50 PM Vegetable Salad, Variety (1 katori)
9:00 PM Linguine Curry (0.75 bowls) Curry Rice
Day 4 of the diet plan for weight loss
Start Day 4 with an egg omelette and a fruit and nut yogurt smoothie.
After that, serve roti, bhindi sabzi, and moong dal.
Steamed rice and palak chole are the last meal of the day.

Day 4 Food Journal
6:30 AM Water with Cucumber for Detox (1 glass)
8:00 AM Smoothie made with yogurt and fruit (0.75 glass)
Omelet with one egg per serving

12:00 PM Slightly Skimmed Paneer (100 grams)
Mixed Vegetable Salad at 2:00 PM (1 katori)
2:10 PM Cooked Green Gram Whole Dal (1 katori)
Bengali sabzi
1 roti and 1 chapati

4:00 PM One orange (2-5/8" diameter) fruit. Buttermilk (1 glass) (1 glass)
5:30 PM less sugar, milk, and coffee (0.5 teacups)
8:50 PM Vegetable Salad, Variety (1 katori)
9:00 PM Chole Palak (1 bowl) Cooked Rice (0.5 katori)
Day 5 of the diet plan for weight loss
On the fifth day, have a cup of skim milk and some pea poha for breakfast.
In the afternoon, have a mission roti with a low-fat paneer dish.
Enjoy roti, curd, and aloo baingan tamatar ki sabzi to cap off the day.

5-Day Diet Chart
6:30 AM Detox Water with Cucumber (1 glass)
8:00 AM Low-Fat Milk (1 glass) Poda Peas (1.5 Katori)
Noon Slightly Skimmed Paneer (100 grams)
2:00 PM Vegetable Salad, Variety (1 katori)
2:10 PM Paneer Curry With Less Fat

4:00 PM (1 cup, 1" chunks) papaya Buttermilk (1 glass) (1 glass)
5:30 PM Tea with Less Milk and Sugar (1 teacup)
8:50 PM Vegetable Salad, Variety (1 katori)
9:00 PM Curd Baingan Tamatar Ki Sabzi Aloo

Day 6 of the diet plan for weight loss
Eat idli with sambar for breakfast and roti with curd and aloo baingan tamatar ki sabzi for lunch on Day 6.
Eat green gram with roti and bhindi sabzi to conclude Day 6.
Chart for diet on day 6
6:30 AM Detox Water with Cucumber (1 glass)
8:00 AM Various Sambar (1 bowl) Idli (2 idli) (2 idli)
Noon Slightly Skimmed Paneer (100 grams)
2:00 PM Vegetable Salad, Variety (1 katori)
2:10 PM Curd Baingan Tamatar Ki Sabzi Aloo
4:00 PM sliced fruit (1 cup) Buttermilk (1 glass) (1 glass)
5:30 PM less sugar, milk, and coffee (0.5 teacups)
8:50 PM Vegetable Salad, Variety (1 katori)
9:00 PM Cooked Green Gram Whole Dal (1 katori) Bengali sabzi

Day 7 of the diet plan for weight loss
Start the seventh day with green garlic chutney and besan chili.
Lunch should consist of steaming rice and palak chole.
Enjoy a missi roti and low-fat paneer stew to end the week on a healthy note.
7-Day Diet Chart
6:30 AM Detox Water with Cucumber (1 glass)

8:00 AM Green garlic chutney and two slices of cheese with besan chilla (3 tablespoons)
Noon Slightly Skimmed Paneer (100 grams)
2:00 PM Vegetable Salad, Variety (1 katori)
2:10 PM Chole Palak (1 bowl) Cooked Rice
4:00 PM 0.5 small (2-3/4" dia.) apples with buttermilk (1 glass)
5:30 PM Tea with Less Milk and Sugar (1 teacup)
8:50 PM Vegetable Salad, Variety (1 katori)
9:00 PM Paneer Curry With Less Fat (1 katori) Ms. Roti Balanced Meal Plans for Losing Weight
Make sure your diet plan is balanced and ensures that you get all the nutrients you need when creating it.

Add the following nutrients to your diet plan as a result:
1. Dietary Plan for Carbohydrates
The majority of the daily calories you need should come from carbohydrates because they are the body's primary energy source. However, it's crucial to pick the proper kind of carbohydrates. Simple carbohydrates, such as bread, biscuits, white rice, and wheat flour, are unhealthy because they are too sweet.

As opposed to simple carbohydrates, choose complex carbs since they are higher in fiber and include more nutrients. This is because complex carbohydrates high in fiber take longer to digest and make you feel fuller for longer, making them the greatest choice for weight management.

Oats, brown rice, and millets like ragi are all excellent sources of complex carbohydrates.

carbohydrates in the finest Indian diet

2. Dietary Proteins

The majority of Indians don't get enough protein each day. This is problematic since the body needs proteins to pump blood and develop and repair tissue, muscles, cartilage, and skin. Hence. A diet rich in protein can also aid in weight loss since it promotes muscle growth, which burns more calories than fat.

For instance, you should include protein in your diet in the form of entire dals, paneer, chana, milk, leafy greens, eggs, white meat, or sprouts, making up roughly 30% of your total calories. Every meal has to include one serving of protein.

protein-rich foods for the ideal Indian diet

3. Diet for Fats
Although they have a poor image, fats are an important dietary category because they help the body create hormones, store vitamins, and provide us energy. One-fifth or 20% of your diet, according to experts, should be made up of polyunsaturated, monounsaturated, and Omega-3 fatty acids.

The best method to ingest fats, for instance, is to use a variety of oils for different meals, such as olive oil, rice bran oil, mustard oil, soya bean, sesame, sunflower, and groundnut oil, along with moderate amounts of butter and ghee. But for a well-balanced Indian diet plan, you must absolutely eliminate trans fats, which are present in fried foods.

optimum Indian dietary oils

4. Nutrients and vitamins Food menu
For the body to operate properly and to promote metabolism, neuron and muscle function, bone maintenance, and cell creation, vitamins A, E, B12, D, calcium, and iron are necessary. Minerals are also present in foods like nuts, oilseeds, fruits, and green leafy vegetables because they are generally sourced from plants, meat, and fish.

Nutritionists and experts advise eating 100 grams of fruits and 100 grams of vegetables each day.

minerals and vitamins in the finest Indian diet plan

5. Meal Substitutions in the Indian Weight Loss Diet
Replace the bad items in your Indian Diet plan with their better equivalents for one of the simplest methods to eat healthily.

For instance, air-popped popcorn instead of potato chips might satisfy your urge for a snack to nibble on.

Therefore, it would be wonderful if you looked into some healthy meal replacement choices that you may attempt in the future.

These routines will assist you in maintaining your health together with a balanced meal plan for weight loss:

Instead of three large meals, try having three smaller meals and a few snack breaks throughout the day in controlled portions. By spreading out your meals at regular intervals, you can avoid bloating and acid reflux while also avoiding hunger pangs. So, give up eating junk food by incorporating healthier snack options into your Indian diet plan.
Eat dinner earlier: Other societies around the world tend to eat dinner later than Indians do. After dinner, metabolism slows down, which can result in weight gain. By 8 p.m., experts advise eating your final meal of the day.

Drink a lot of water:
How can increasing your water intake assist in weight loss? First off, there are no calories in it. A glass of water might also help quell hunger cravings. To lose weight, drink six to eight glasses of water every day. You can also discover a list of beverages that can aid in weight loss here.

Eat plenty of fiber: Fiber helps with digestion and heart health, so an individual needs at least 15 gm of it daily.

Some excellent sources of fiber include apples, broccoli, lentils, flax seeds, and lentils.